Homemade Lotion Bars
30 Natural Lotion Bars Recipes

Table of Contents:

Introduction: Forget all About Store-Bought! 3

Chapter 1: Oil Based Bar Lotion 4

Chapter 2: Organic Lotion Bars for your Pets!..16

Chapter 3: Organic Lotion Bars for Health and Beauty 24

Chapter 4: Other Uses for Organic Bars 32

Conclusion: Why I DIY my own Organic Lotion Bars...37

Introduction: Forget all About Store-Bought!

Once you start making your own organic lotion bars there is really no end to what you can do with them. They are healthy and they are convenient. With fragrance and healthy vitamins and minerals packed into something the size and shape of a bar of soap. They are also rather easy to make.

Just put the ingredients together and sit it out at room temperature until the bars become solid. I absolutely promise you, when you know how to make your own organic lotion bars you will never go back to the store-bought variety ever again!

Chapter 1: Oil Based Bar Lotion

In this chapter we will run through the best organic lotion bars that an oil base can provide.

Chocolate Organic Bar

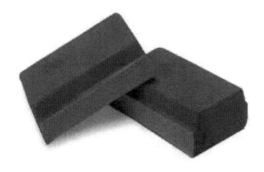

Who doesn't like chocolate? Well, in this refreshing bar with a splash of coconut and olive oil, you can have it!

Here are the exact ingredients:
12 oz coconut oil
50 oz olive oil
6 oz cocoa butter
32 oz cold water

To get started take out a medium sized mixing bowl and add 3 teaspoons of cocoa powder followed by the coconut and olive oil. Vigorously stir these ingredients together. Next pour your mixture into a bar mold.

Peach and Almond Oil Soap

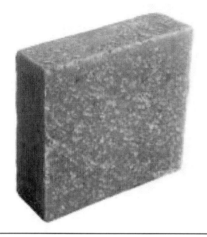

Well isn't that just peachy! With this Peach and Almond Soap the aroma is incredible! And with the hint of soybean oil that makes up this organic bar's ingredients, this organic lotion bar works as an excellent exfoliant and with just a few lathers your skin is incredibly refreshed!

Here are the exact ingredients:
30 oz soybean oil
14 oz palm oil
12oz coconut oil
7 oz almond oil
3 cups water

Take out a large saucepan, toss in your 3 cups of cold water. Set your burner to high. Now add all of your oil ingredients and continually stir the mixture while it boils. After 5 minutes of boiling pour the contents of the pan into your bar mold. Now let sit in mold for 22 hours.

Organic Veggie Bar Lotion

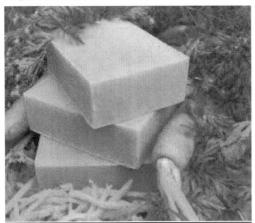

This organic lotion bar provides you with an all natural way to clean up! With a vegetable oil base, this exfoliating bar cleans and moisturizes with just a few refreshing lathers!

Here are the exact ingredients:

22 oz coconut oil
22 oz olive oil
18 oz canola oil
18 oz vegetable oil
4 cups water

Put your 4 cups of water in a medium sauce pan an set your burner to high. Dump in your oil ingredients, boil for 10 minutes. Now dump the blended ingredients into your mold and allow it to solidify for about 15 hours.

Coconut Oil Organic Bar Lotion

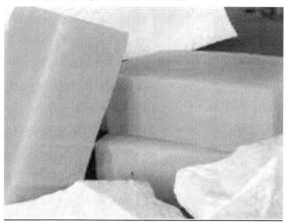

This soap is very smooth and gentle to the touch. Great for sensitive skin!

Here are the exact ingredients:

78 oz olive oil

6 oz coconut oil

6 oz palm oil

4 cups water

Mix your ingredients together in a mixing bowl and then dump then into a large saucepan. Boil well for 20 minutes and then dispense into your mold. Allow bars to solidify for at least 22 hours.

Soft and Silky Milk Bar Lotion

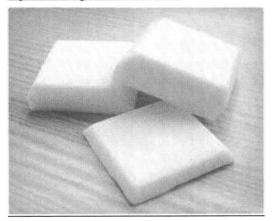

It's Milky and its Silky with a hint of dark Olive Oil!

Here are the exact ingredients:

1 cup vegetable shortening

14 oz dark olive oil

15 oz safflower oil

5 cups milk

10 oz lye

1 oz Borax

2 tablespoons honey

2 trays ice cubes

First melt your cup of veggie shortening in a medium saucepan followed by your safflower and olive oil. Next grab a medium sized plastic container and fill it half full with water.

Now dump your 2 trays of ice cubes into the container. Now pour about a saucepan full of cold milk into the container followed by your 10 ounces of lye. Stir this mixture together for about 10 minutes.

Now dump the contents of your plastic container into your saucepan of oil. Follow this, by adding your borax and honey to the pan. Stir this together for a few minutes and then dump the entire contents into a blender.

Set your blender for "Whip and allow the ingredients to blend for about 2 minutes on this setting. Finally, after everything is blended, add the mixture to your bar mold and after about 22 hours it should solidify and be ready to go!

Lavender Oil Organic Bar Lotion

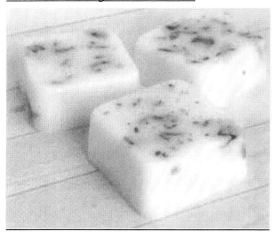

Using the best of essential lavender oil, this bar lotion is as soothing as it gets!

Here are the exact ingredients:
1 tablespoon coconut oil
1 tablespoon palm oil
2 tablespoons olive oil
4 tablespoons lavender oil
2 tablespoons almond oil
3 cups milk

Mix oils together in a medium saucepan on high heat. Now add milk to the pan and stir the mixture for about 15 minutes. Once you've done this you can then pour your mix into your molds and after 20 hours you have yourself another great batch of organic lotion bars!

Castor Oil and Yogurt Organic Lotion Bar

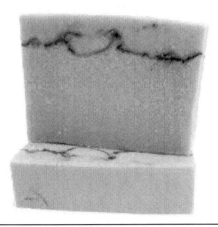

This organic lotion bar contains nothing but the best! The fragrance is great and the effect it has on your skin is even better!

Here are the exact ingredients:

17 oz coconut oil

20 oz olive oil

20 oz palm oil

7 oz palm kernel oil

10 oz lye

3 cups water

17 oz yogurt

7 oz castor oil

3 oz avocado oil

First off take your lye and add it to a bowl filled with your 3 cups of water. Put this away for the moment and then place a saucepan on medium heat and add all of your oil ingredients.

While your oils are melting, then place your yogurt in a container and heat in the microwave for about 55 seconds. Now blend your lye mix with the oils and then finally, add the yogurt to the mix. Now pour the contents of the saucepan into the mold and let it sit for about 20 hours or until sufficiently hardened.

Honey Bee Sudsy Soap Organic Bar

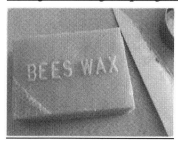

With an eye catching and Earthy brown color, this soap is as sweet as honey!

Here are the exact ingredients:

12 oz vegetable shortening

4 oz coconut oil

1 oz bees wax

2 cups water

1 oz lye

Mix all of your oil ingredients into a medium sauce pan on high heat with your 2 cups of water. Now set this aside so that it can cool.

After this, pour your vegetable shortening and lye into the pan and stir vigorously. Now add your bees wax and blend together well for about 5 minutes. Just pour this mix into your molds, let it sit out for about 32 hours and you are done!

Deluxe Olive Oil Organic Bar Lotion

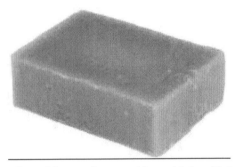

Olive Oil is great for your skin, and infused into this beautiful lotion bar it is even better!

Here are the exact ingredients:

2 oz olive oil

3 cups water

6 ounces of lye

Take out a medium sized mixing bowl and add your water, lye, and olive oil. Now blend it all together until it is nice and thick. Pour this into your mold and let it sit for about 22 hours and this organic lotion bar is complete!

Banana Oil Organic Bar

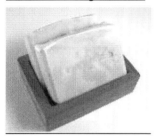

I love bananas and I love them even more now that I can have them as an organic lotion bar!

Here are the exact ingredients:
40 ounces vegetable shortening
10 ounces olive oil
10 ounces canola oil
2 cups cold milk
10 ounces lye
4 ounces whipped cream
10 ounces banana oil
1 banana
4 tablespoons critic acid
4 tablespoons sugar

Combine your oils together in a pan and place on a burner set to medium. After your oils melt together turn off your burner and put the pan away for the moment. Now take your citric acid, banana, and cream and put them in a blender. Blend for about 15 minutes. Now fill sink with water dump your ice and pour your milk into the sink. Follow this by mixing your sugar into the ice milk water. Now you can dump the lye into the mix, stir well and let all of this sit for about 20 minutes. Put this mixture into your blender and mix together on its lowest setting for two minutes. Dump your blended ingredients into your molding and allow it to solidify for about 22 hours.

Sunflower Oil Organic Bar Lotion

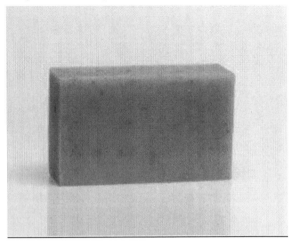

This organic bar soap is so good it is almost edible! With its wholesome sunflower oil, oatmeal, and honey ingredients, it is a real treat for your skin too!

Here are the exact ingredients:

34 oz olive oil

2 oz castor oil

2 oz coconut oil

2 oz sunflower oil

2 oz cocoa butter

4 oz lye

18 oz buttermilk

9 oz distilled water

1 cup oatmeal

1 cup honey

Take out a crock pot and add your oils on a low heat setting. Now take your water and buttermilk cubes and add them together in a mixing bowl. Now go to your sink and add your water and ice.

This should be followed by your addition of lye to the mix. After a few moments take this mixture and add it to your oils in the crock pot.

Finally add your honey and oatmeal. After about 20 minutes you can then fill up your molds. Allow another 22 hours for it to solidify and your Sunflower Oil Organic Bar Lotions is complete!

Chapter 2: Organic Lotion Bars for your Pets!

Every dog has his day right? Well, now he can have his lotion too! Check out these great organic lotion bar recipes for your pets!

Smelly Doggy Organic Bar Lotion

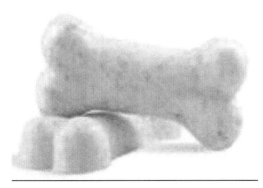

An organic lotion bar for that doggy of yours who could use a little odor adjustment!

Here are the exact ingredients:

7 oz water

3 oz full fat buttermilk

4 oz lye

5 oz coconut oil

7 oz palm oil

7 oz olive oil

7 oz soybean oil

2 oz neem oil

1 oz of rosemary essential oil

To get going on this doggy recipe take your water and add your lye. Once you've done this set it aside to cool. Combine with buttermilk. Now begin melting your oil in the microwave, after you've done this add them to your slow cooker. Place your milk/water, and lye in this mix. Now add your rosemary and neem. Stir well and deposit in your molds to make your organic lotion bars. Let set for about 22 hours.

Fruit Dog Organic Bar Lotion

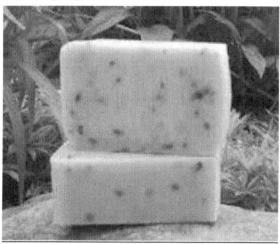

Your doggy will smell really good with this one!

Here are the exact ingredients:

72 ounces olive oil

12 ounces coconut oil

22ounces cold distilled water

10 ounces lye

1 sweet orange essential oil

1 ounce citronella essential oil

2 tablespoons orange peel

First combine your coconut and olive oil in a large saucepan and momentarily put it to the side. Next shred your orange peel and place it in a mixing bowl. After this add your eucalyptus, citronella, and sweet orange essential oils.

Once you've done this take out another bowl add water to it, and then deposit your lye into the bowl. Mix well for a few moments. Next, go back to your stove and turn on your burner heating up your oils. Dump the lye water mixture into the pan and stir well. Do this for about 45 minutes until all ingredients are thoroughly blended together.

Now add in your orange peel and other ingredients and stir vigorously for about 5 additional minutes. Dump the entire contents of your pan into your molds, leave to solidify for about 35 hours and soon your doggy will be smelling very fruity indeed!

Creamy Organic Cat Bar

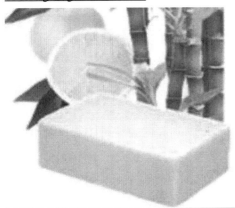

It may not be catnip but your feline friends are going to just love this one!

Here are the exact ingredients:

1 cup Shea butter

1 cup beeswax

2 tablespoons coconut oil

2 cups water

Mix these three main ingredients together in a medium mixing bowl and then dump the entire contents of the bowl into a medium saucepan filled with your 2 cups of water. Stir vigorously until smooth. Now just pour your mixture into your bar mold and wait about 12 hours for it to solidify and you are done.

Happy Paws Organic Lotion Bar

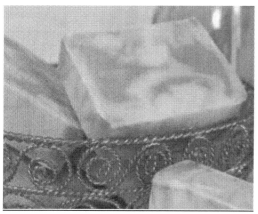

Even our pets can have sensitive skin, but one whiff of these lotion bars and they'll be happy!

Here are the exact ingredients:

7 oz cocoa butter

7 oz Shea butter

7 oz beeswax

7 oz olive butter

7 oz avocado oil

1 oatmeal colloidal

To kick this DIY off right you are going to need a medium sized saucepan. Place it on medium heat and toss in your 7 ounces of Beeswax, Cocoa Butter, Shea Butter, and Olive Butter. Stir vigorously until it is all well blended together. Now add in your colloidal oatmeal and keep stirring the contents until it thoroughly dissolves into the mix. Now simply pour the contents of your pan into your molding and let sit out for about 18 hours to harden. Your pet will thank you for it!

Organic Flea Shampoo Bar

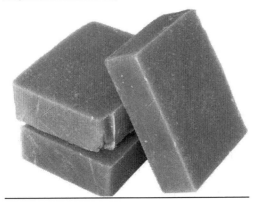

Ok! I know that it is not quite so pleasant to talk about, but every good dog owner knows that a flea repellant shampoo bar is a great necessity for keeping their little doggy flea free!

Here are the exact ingredients

1 cup of coconut oil

½ cup of mango butter

½ cup of beeswax

¼ cup of dried rosemary leaves

1 teaspoon of dried whole cloves

2 tablespoons of dried or fresh thyme

½ teaspoon of cinnamon powder

¼ cup of dried catnip leaf

Fill a small saucepan with water and put it on a burner set to high. Now put your cloves, thyme, cinnamon, dried rosemary, mint and catnip in the pan. Boil these ingredients together for about half an hour. Now add your cup of coconut oil, half a cup of mango butter, and half a cup of beeswax, stir thoroughly until thick. Dump the contents of the pan into your bar molds and your naturally made, organic flea shampoo bar is ready for service!

Organic Shiny Dog Coat Bar

Your dog deserves a soft, shiny coat, and this organic bar promises to deliver. And as an added bonus, the ingredients of this bar also serve as a proactive and natural bug repellant!

Here are the exact ingredients:
1 cup of beeswax
1 cup of cocoa butter
½ cup of organic coconut oil
½ cup castor oil
11 drops citronella oil
11 drops eucalyptus oil
11 drops clove oil
7 drops peppermint oil

Take out your beeswax, castor oil, and coconut oil and dump them into a medium sauce pan, allowing the ingredients to melt on high heat. Now stir in your drops of citronella oil, eucalyptus oil, clove oil, and peppermint oil.

Once these are all boiled together, take the pan off the burner and allow the contents to cool off for about 5 minutes. Finally, just dump the contents out into your molding and your Organic Shiny Dog Coat bar is complete!

Organic Mosquito Bar Lotion

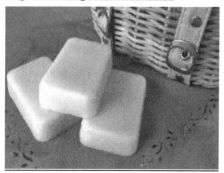

This summer the mosquito's were atrocious, and they are predicted to be even worse next year, so what can we do to protect our pets? We can use this specialty organic Mosquito Bar Lotion of course!

Here are the exact ingredients:
1 tablespoon of beeswax
5 tablespoons of Shea butter
3 tablespoons of coconut oil
11 drops of Miracle Grow oil
11 drops of citronella oil
4 drops of peppermint essential oil
22 drops of lemongrass essential oil
3 of cups of water

Dump your 3 cups of water in a large saucepan and place it on a burner set for medium heat. Add all of the above mentioned ingredients. Boil for 20 minutes while vigorously stirring. Allow the contents to blend together until it has a thickened texture.

Now simply fill your mold casings with the liquid. Allow these bars to solidify over the next 12 hours and your Organic Mosquito Bar Lotion is ready keep those pesky mosquitoes at bay!

Chapter 3: Organic Lotion Bars for Health and Beauty

You don't have to go to bed, bath, and beyond in order to have good products for health and beauty. In this chapter let's go over some of the best organic lotion bars for enhancing appearance and overall wellness.

Organic Shampoo Bar Lotion

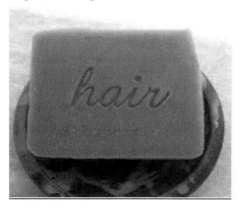

It's like a bar of soap but you use it on your head!

Here are the exact ingredients:

8 oz coconut oil

8 oz olive oil

4 oz castor oil

2 oz jojoba oil

1 oz Shea butter

1 oz cocoa butter

1 oz beeswax

2 cups water

4 oz coconut milk

2 oz lye

First off, place your coconut milk and 2 cups of water into a mixing bowl. Now add your lye and stir the ingredients together thoroughly. After you've done this, set the bowl to the side and then in a medium sized sauce pan add your oils.

Turn the burner on high and allow all of the oil ingredients to melt together for about 5 minutes. Then turn off your burner and dump the oils from your pan into a crock pot and place the crock pot's heat on low.

Now add your other ingredients to the mix and stir vigorously in the crock pot for about ten minutes. Once the mixture has thickened, go ahead and put the lid on your crock pot and let the entire contents heat up for about 2 hours.

Once your 2 hours are up, go ahead and turn off your crock pot and pour the blended ingredients into your bar molds. All you have to do now is wait 12 hours for the bars to harden and your organic shampoo bar lotion is ready to go.

Energizing Hot Pepper Bar

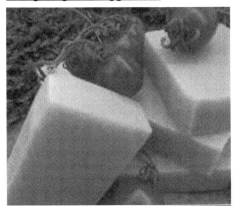

Utilizing the kick of some hot peppers, this organic bar lotion will help refresh your senses and get your day started!

Here are the exact ingredients:
4 oz avocado oil

24 oz coconut oil

28 oz olive oil

4 oz castor oil

2 oz mango butter

9 oz lye

3 cups water

2 dry mint leaves

Lay your 2 dry mint leaves at the bottom of a medium sized mixing bowl and then dump 3 cups of water over the leaves. Now pour hot water over these leaves to infuse the mint into the water.

Place this bowl to the side for now allowing it to continue taking in this mint ingredient. Now go to a medium sauce pan placed on high heat and add the rest of your ingredients. While the contents of the pan begins to boil, vigorously stir the ingredients together, let them cook together for another 15 to 20 minutes.

Once you've done this pour the contents of your mixing bowl into your pan and stir it together with your oils. Allow all of these ingredients to cook for another 10 minutes before turning off the burner.

Now let the pan cool off for 5 minutes and then dump the contents into the bar molding. Wait about 12 to 15 hours for your bar to solidify and your energizing hot pepper bar is complete.

Organic Massage Bar

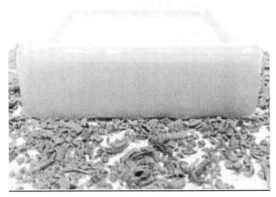

We could all use a massage sometimes right? So what better than one that comes with an exfoliating punch like this one? You have just got to check out the Organic Massage Bar!

Here are the exact ingredients:
2 tablespoons cocoa butter
1 tablespoon Shea butter
1 tablespoon safflower oil
4 drops lavender oil
4 drops rose germanium oil

To begin, take your cocoa butter and all of your oil ingredients and melt them together in a medium saucepan on medium heat.

Once everything melts together take the pan off of the burner. Stir these ingredients well and then dispense into your bar molds and let it solidify over the next 24 hours. Your Silky Lotion Massage Bar is now ready to give you the massage of your life!

Citrus and Herbs Exfoliating Organic Bar Lotion

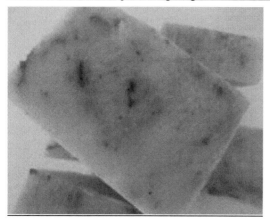

With its citrus blend, this soap is a great way to clean and exfoliate your face!

Here are the exact ingredients:

11 oz palm oil

11 oz coconut oil

11 oz olive oil

4 oz cocoa butter

5 oz Lye

2 cups water

Put your water in a medium sauce pan and put the burner on high. Now add all of the ingredients except for the lye. Allow your ingredients to boil while stirring vigorously.

Now finally, after about 5 minutes add your lye to the mix and continuing stirring for another few minutes. Once all of the ingredients are nice and thick turn off the butter and pour the contents of your pan into your bar molds.

Organic Lemon Balm Lotion

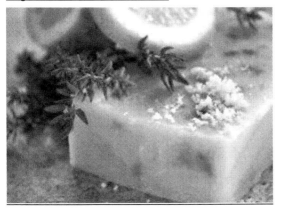

For a great, refreshing organic bar with lemon zest, try out this organic lotion bar!

Here are the exact ingredients:

1 cup goat's milk

5 drops lemon oil

1 oz Dried Lemon

Get out a medium sized mixing bowl and mix all of the ingredient together. Now put your 2 cups of water in a saucepan on medium heat. Dump the contents of your mixing bowl into the sauce pan.

Stir until the mixture boils and thickens. Turn off your burn and let the ingredients cool off for 20 minutes. Pour the contents into your molding and let it solidify for at least 10 hours.

Organic Potassium Moisturizing Bar

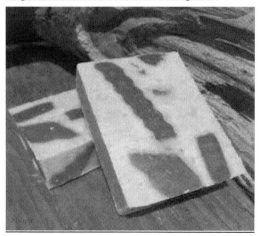

This organic bar lotion is easy on the eyes and even easier on the pores as a great moisturizer.

Here are the exact ingredients:

17 oz olive oil

8 oz coconut oil

7 oz potassium hydroxide

22 ounces filtered water

3 ounces borax

First put your 17 ounces of olive oil and your 8 ounces of coconut oil in a slow cooker and put the heat on its lowest setting. Now add your potassium hydroxide to the mixture, slowly stirring it in. After this add your 22 ounces of filtered water. Now stir your mixture continually for about 10 minutes.

Once you've done this add your 3 ounces of borax, shut the lid of the slow cooker and let it cook for another 30 minutes. When your 30 minutes is up, turn the cooker off and let it cool down for another 15 minutes. Now you can scoop out the contents of the slow cooker and deposit them into your bar molds. Let the mixture sit in the molds for about 22 hours.

Organic Lotion Bar for Shaving

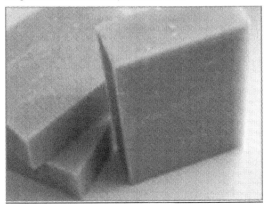

We gotta shave right? Well why not shave in style with this organic wonder?

Here are the exact ingredients:
18 oz palm kernel oil
18 oz coconut oil
38 oz buttermilk
10 oz lye

In a medium sauce pan add your oils, boil them on high heat. Now add your buttermilk and lye stirring them vigorously into the mix for about 10 minutes. Turn off your burner and let the ingredients cool for 10 more minutes. Now dump the contents into the molding and after 22 hours your Organic Lotion Bar for Shaving will be ready to rock and roll!

Chapter 4: Other Uses for Organic Bars

For our last chapter in this book lets go over some of the other uses and novelties for organic bar lotion that may often be over looked, but are nonetheless worthwhile.

Organic Beer Bar

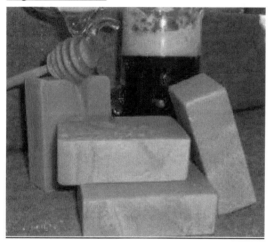

There can be only one; Organic Beer Bar!

Here are the exact ingredients:
22 ounces of coconut oil
22 ounces of olive oil
37 ounces of flat beer
10 ounces of lye

To begin, put a large saucepan on the burner and set it to medium heat. Now put your coconut oil, olive oil, and beer into the pan. Stir well and let this mixture boil for about 5 minutes. Now add your lye to the mixture and stirring it in vigorously as it dissolves into the rest of the ingredients. After about 5 more minutes take the pan off the burner and let the mixture cool off for a few moments. Finally add the whole mixture to the mold casings and once the soap solidifies your Organic Beer Bar is ready.

Organic Soda Soap

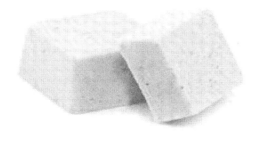

Now that we have covered the beer; how about some soda? Try some organic soda soap.

Here are the exact ingredients:
3 cups of Sprite
4 cups of water
1 cup of lime juice
4 ounces of borax

First dump your four cups of water into a medium sauce pan and set the burner to high. Once the water is boiling go ahead and add your four cups of Sprite, followed by your cup of lime juice. Stir these ingredients thoroughly for about 10 minutes.

Now turn your burner off and add your 4 ounces of borax, stir again for a few more minutes until the ingredients have a thick consistency and texture. Let the mixture cool for a few minutes and then dispense the liquid into the bar molds. It will generally take about 15 hours for this mix to solidify. Enjoy!

Iodine Organic Bar Lotion

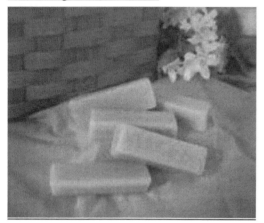

This kind of organic bar lotion may be less well known but it serves a great use. As a completely organic bar of iodine, just by rubbing this lotion on your cuts, scrapes, and other injuries it disinfects the wound.

Here are the ingredients:
1 cup of water
1 ounce of iodine
2 ounces of olive oil
5 ounces of milk

Put a small sauce pan on high heat and add your cup of water. Let the water boil for about 10 minutes and then add in your olive oil and milk stirring the mixture in for another 5 minutes.

Now turn your burner off and add your ounce of iodine. Mix thoroughly and then pour into your bar mold. Let it solidify over the next 22 hours, then take it out and store it somewhere you will really need it. I always keep my own bar of organic iodine lotion in a first aid kit.

Organic Strawberry Bar Lotion

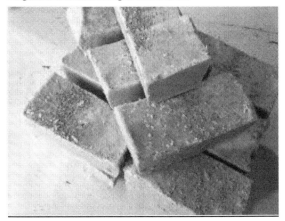

As good as a bunch of fresh picked strawberries, this soothing organic bar lotion will have you feeling and smelling great!

Here are the exact ingredients:

2 cups water

4 oz sodium hydroxide flakes

8 oz coconut oil

7 oz palm oil

2.3 oz avocado butter

5 oz macadamia nut oil

2 oz castor oil

2 teaspoons spinach powder

2 teaspoons rose kaolin clay

1 oz fresh picked strawberry

Take a mixing bowl and add your water and lye, gently mixing them together. Put this to the side and then in a separate container add all of your other ingredients together and then cook in the microwave for 45 seconds (or until melted).

Now take both of your bowls of ingredients and combine them into a medium sauce pan on high heat. Once you have done this, you can add your Rose Kolin Clay. Boil and stir for ten minutes. Allow to cool and pour into your bar mold.

Organic Goat Milk Lotion Bar

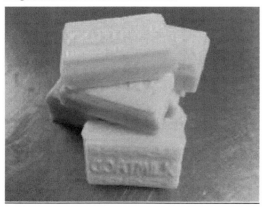

Goat's Milk? A little bit unusual maybe, but great for your complexion!

Here are the exact ingredients:

7 oz beeswax

3 oz coconut oil

3 oz hemp seed oil

3 oz jojoba oil

3 oz hemp seed butter

1 tablespoon goat's milk powder

1 oz honey almond

Put your beeswax in a medium saucepan on low heat. Now deposit your hemp butter and your goat's milk powder; stir until well blended. Next, add in all of your oils and thoroughly mix them as well. Let this boil together for 5 minutes. Now simply dump the contents of the pan into your mold and let solidify for about 24 hours.

Conclusion: Why I DIY my own Organic Lotion Bars

It was just a few years ago that I found myself making my first Organic Bar Lotion. We had just started the fall season in early October when I started seeing pumpkin based products every time I turned around. This theme continued during my job site's office party later that month. But it was something one of my coworkers had brought that really caught my eye.

As a gift at our get together she had passed out homemade "pumpkin spice organic soap". The soap appeared to be very well done and smelled incredible. I thought they were fantastic, so I asked her where she bought these lovely toiletries.

That's when she informed me that she made them herself. This piqued my interest, and as soon as I came home I researched how to make Organic Lotion Bars and I have been hooked ever since. I hope that this book has been helpful and enjoyable. Thank you!

FREE Bonus Reminder

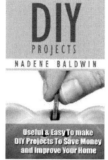

If you have not grabbed it yet, please go ahead and download your special bonus report *"DIY Projects. 13 Useful & Easy To Make DIY Projects To Save Money & Improve Your Home!"*
Simply Click the Button Below

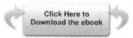

OR **Go to This Page**
http://diyhomecraft.com/free

BONUS #2: More Free & Discounted Books or Products
Do you want to receive more Free/Discounted Books or Products?
We have a mailing list where we send out our new Books or Products when they go free or with a discount on Amazon. Click on the link below to sign up for Free & Discount Book & Product Promotions.
=> Sign Up for Free & Discount Book & Product Promotions <=

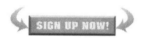

OR Go to this URL
http://zbit.ly/1WBb1Ek

Made in the USA
Middletown, DE
15 February 2023

24924258R00022